Can a vagina really buy a Mercedes?

What can your pelvic floor do for you?

by
Jenni Russell

First printed in Great Britain in 2005 by
JM Print Services Ltd
Registered Office:
90 Plumstead High Street
London SE18 1SL

email: jmprintservices@ntlworld.com

Copyright © Jenni Russell 2004

Published by Jenni Russell

Printed and Bound in Great Britain by
JM Print Services Ltd, Essex

The moral right of the author has been asserted.

All rights reserved. Without limiting the rights under copyright reserved above, no part of this publicaton may be reproduce, stored or introduced into a retrieval system, or transmitted, in any form or by any means (electronic, mechanical, photocopying, recording or otherwise), without the prior written permission of both the copyright owner and the publisher of this book.

A catalogue record for this book will be available from the British Library.

ISBN 0-9551333-0-0

In loving memory of Aunty Norma, I finished the book.

To my boogie dance partner Lee Roy July - I will realize my dream and hopefully Lee I can get to commission and realize yours.

Contents

Foreword	2
Preface	3
Introduction	4
Wet or dry? (an incontinence issue)	9
Awakening our 'core' - Discovering our trump card!	12
So what's so special about our Pelvic Floor?	25
Awakening the Pelvic Floor	29
Along came Gynaflex	44
Conclusion	47
Glossary	49
References and further reading	52
About the author	53
Special thanks	55

Foreword

We live in a world of multiple puzzles and paradoxes. One such paradox you are sure to be familiar with is that of advanced technology in science and medicine (Evolution) coupled with the obvious loss of health, vitality and physical function and beauty of our bodies (De-evolution). The core of our Body, being the core of our Being, reflects not only the true functionality of our inner life, but often our outer life as well.

The pelvic girdle is the interface between our rhythmic and metabolic systems and our legs or lower limb system. The functionality of this metabolic, rhythmic, limb system greatly impacts our mobility, our sexuality and our physical beauty.

In this beautiful little book, Jenni has given you useful exercises for improving this all-important pelvic interface, which joins our inner and outer worlds. If you follow her approach you will certainly enjoy both improved functionality and a better sex life. This effort will be rewarding, for it affords freedom of the Soul.

Paul Chek, H.H.P.
Founder CHEK Institute
Vista, CA

www.chekinstitute.com

Preface

This book is meant to be entertaining, and educational. In the following chapters we will look at the issue of lower abdominals and pelvic floor and their affects on incontinence and sexual function. I have added humour to a very taboo subject. Many women suffer silently with mild bladder weakness, or sexual dysfunction because they are too embarrassed to admit that something as simple as a joke could cause discomfort when they laugh, or that their pelvic floor is so de-conditioned that they do not have any great sexual experience because they cannot feel anything. Let us use the information in this book to redress this issue. The dialogue is user friendly. I have broken down the science, no dictionary needed here. The cartoon sketches add humour, the diagrams for the exercises give a visual indication of what to do and the wording is relative. Use the Glossary at the back of the book to help understand any technical terms used.

Introduction

For many years, as part of my aerobic and conditioning classes, I have taught my clients the importance of the pelvic floor muscles and their relationship with a good sex life. I thank a dear friend for this, for he had an experience after his fiancé had their baby. "My god Jenni, now I know what they mean when they say it's like dipping your wick in a well"! Until that day fifteen years ago I never ever thought about the importance of my vaginal wall and its 'tightness'. That wasn't me. Having discussed this issue with my girlfriends we decided we would rather be a part of the club I named the 'Pinhead Posse' – meaning that the vaginal opening would be the size of a pinhead figuratively speaking. I would never want to guess whether or not my partner was inside me after childbirth. I would always want to feel him, so a de-conditioned and stretched vaginal wall would not allow this to be. I wanted to have an enjoyable and active sex life way into retirement - so having a baby at age 31 and then wondering what was happening down there could only lead to 40 years of torture and an eventual loss of my sexual desire. Sex, in my opinion, is as important to women as it is to men – we're just not as greedy!

I went on to devise some crazy ways of doing pelvic floor exercises at various

Introduction

speeds, in different positions, and to music to make it fun, but also to give people ideas of how to work it into their bedrooms. I have spoken in jest at dinner parties with close friends and their husbands, and then they had tried these things at home with him saying: "You're doing Jenni's stuff aren't you"? It was working! Men would tell their women to keep coming to class because it was having positive effects aesthetically and sexually.

At this point, we had given no thought or paid any attention to the relationship of the pelvic floor and incontinence as no one complained about leaking. The courses of old qualified you to teach exercise to music or, gym instruction and circuits. (Pre-Natal touched on this briefly). Never mentioned, so never thought about.

Then, four and a half years ago, I was introduced to Swiss Ball Training at a private health club where I work, and the person I refer to as 'the guru of Swiss Ball and Kinesiology' - Paul Chek. (A person, I sincerely respect and admire). This course was to change the way I trained, and without realizing, changed my sex life and how I would teach pelvic floor exercise.

Introduction

My next course with Paul Chek (C.H.E.K. Institute) was Scientific Core Conditioning - a course focusing on all the muscles of the abdominal structure and those of the back and neck that relate to it. There are three main parts: the upper Abdominals (Rectus), the waistline (Oblique) and the Low Abdominals (Transversus). The key one is the Transversus. These muscles are the deepest of the tummy muscles behind the belly button.

The course notes under transverses said: "This muscle needs to be activated before we have "full" function of our pelvic floor. This muscle coupled with the multifidus - (a tiny muscle just at the base of our lower back under what we call the erector spine is the true stabilizer for the low back) - and our pelvic floor are fed by the same signal from the brain - (a neurological loop)". When I read this I thought "yeah right"! I had been training for 28 years and had won the title of Britain's Fittest Woman (British Ultrafit Challenge) on three occasions without ever having used this muscle. Friends and partners had been very happy using their pelvic floor independent of this muscle without any complaints. Nonsense was my response. I chose to ignore it.

I found the Swiss Ball fascinating and after watching the high performance

> "Men would tell their women to keep coming to class because it was having positive effects, both aesthetically and sexually"

Introduction

video I decided this was for me. I spent a year developing my lower abdominals as the stabilizers they are and introducing them into all my exercises. I undid all the faulty training patterns and started over again. If I had won national titles without this muscle – my 'powerhouse' – then what would I achieve with it switched on? (I was single at this point). A year passed...

Whilst out on business one evening I met a very charming man. We dated a while and then we had sex. Now if I were a smoker, then I would have had a cigarette! What did this man have that no other partner seemed to

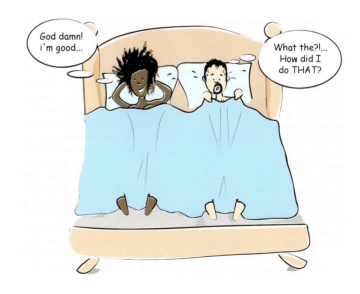

Introduction

possess? He was not well endowed, he was not physically fine tuned, but he did blow me away! I will not deny that we had great chemistry, but alas this relationship did not last. Later that year, I revisited an old boyfriend and low and behold I had the same wild experience I had not previously had with him. I then realized - it was me! My goodness, I had married my lower abdominals with my pelvic floor but as I was single this was the only 'exercise' I had yet to co-ordinate.

'Pinhead Posse' status had finally been reached! I believe now that this magnificent tool, our vagina, that we as women are blessed with can open and close for business, can negotiate all kinds of things from our husbands, change so much that goes on in the bedroom (or any other room in the house) and can give a whole new meaning to how many women view sex or lovemaking. Can a vagina really buy a Mercedes? Many of my friends say, "Yes it can"!

> "If I had won national titles without this muscle – my 'powerhouse' – then what would I achieve with it switched on?"

Wet or dry? (an incontinence issue)

Chapter 1

For many of us women this is a burning question. Shit hot body and 'wet knickers' or shit hot body and 'dry knickers'? Incontinence is a common problem amongst many women whether or not they have had children! Many situations are responsible for this growing issue – and Tenalady continence pads are making some good money because a lot of us are too embarrassed to admit it. (See Chapter 3 for more about this issue).

So what is it that makes us wet ourselves laughing, literally? After all, that is supposed to be a figure of speech! Why is it that for many of us we really do 'lie back and think of England' simply because we are wondering whether or not he is inside us yet? Yes I am hearing some of you – "find a man with a bigger ******" – but if your vaginal wall is like the Blackwall Tunnel then you need to be thinking of narrowing the lanes!

Many women hate exercise. I should know! As a personal trainer I train many women who only exercise as a means to an end, but hate every minute of it. Yet our bodies demand that we exert ourselves daily. The pelvic floor is a bag of muscles. In order for them to work efficiently they need a workout too. Put it this way, "Your body displays the

Wet or dry? (an incontinence issue)

Chapter 1

respect/regard you give/have for it". This muscle although hidden responds to the way it is looked after. Like all other muscles of the body it will either do its job to support and increase blood flow to the area, or not, dependent on its condition.

Food is energy intake and in order for us to not become apples or pears with arms and legs sticking out we need to expend some of that energy, otherwise we will wear it. Metabolism does not get a workout unless you give it one!

It is now time for us women to really take charge of our bodies and realize that this here Vagina is like a diamond -

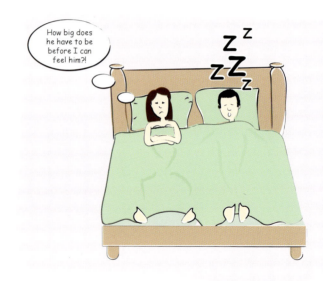

Wet or dry? (an incontinence issue)

Chapter 1

> The pelvic floor is a bag of muscles, and in order for them to work efficiently they need a workout too

precious and to be cherished. After all, it is the canal for which 'life' is bought into this world - there is nothing more precious than that!

It can save us from many embarrassing situations and get us just about anything we really want and not ruin those lovely 'La Perla' underwear we save so hard to buy or receive from our partners as gifts. Think of it this way - 'La Perla' and 'Tenalady,' continence pads' were just not designed to be worn together!

"What do I need to do"? I hear you ask. I want you to be able to read this book, laugh and keep your knickers dry. Firstly, you are going to need to know what/where your 'core' is and the vital relationship it has to 'full' pelvic floor function. Then you are going to need to get to know the muscles in the vagina that are responsible for keeping those knickers dry and those that are responsible for working on that new car! Co-ordination is where the fun comes in.

Read on.

Awakening our 'core' – Discovering our trump card!

Chapter 2

Our transversus abdominals (TVA - our core) are a vital set of muscles we need to get to know. Everything we do emanates from here and these deep abdominal muscles lying behind the belly button are important for everyday wellbeing, posture, movement, protection, central nervous system function, as well as incontinence and enjoyment or sexual satisfaction. Its job is to stabilize the back for which it plays possibly the most important role, whilst generating the movement from the arms and the legs and is the cylinder wall to our pelvic floor.

The Lower Abdominals (Transversus), pelvic floor and a small muscle buried just above the base of lower back (multifidus) share the same neurological loop or fire wire (fed by the same signal from the brain). If our lower abdominals are not switched on then we will never have full function of the pelvic floor or multifidus. (Ref: Scientific Core Conditioning - Paul Chek C.H.E.K. Institute).

Think of the lower abdominals as the middle of a cylinder - the walls of a can, with the diaphragm as the ceiling and the pelvic floor as the base. Now if we have no use for our transversus then our cylinder walls are weak and if the pelvic floor is weak, the result will be a load pushed down from the ceiling (the

> "If our lower abdominals are not switched on then we will never have full function of the pelvic floor or multifidus"

Awakening our 'core' — Discovering our trump card!

Chapter 2

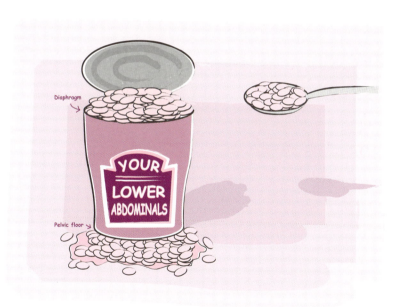

diaphragm) onto/through the pelvic floor without the cylinder wall stopping it. Over time everything that goes in will start/try to push out the bottom. This is more apparent when upper abdominals are overworked and then you do anything load bearing as in running/jumping. If you go to seek medical advice for a weak pelvic floor many medical professionals will get you to work the floor independently of all other muscles and yet nothing in the body works on its own. So if you work this muscle on its own without assistance from the lower abs you have left your ceiling without the support to hold it up and away from the base.

Awakening our 'core' – Discovering our trump card!

Chapter 2

Over time the contents become too much for the base and, either it begins to seep or it gives way!

What we need to do is learn how to 'awaken and switch on' our lower abdominals. We need to learn how to co-ordinate limb movement whilst stabilizing our trunks and then learn how to 'switch on' our pelvic floor, coordinating all three together. We then learn which parts of the vagina are vital to closing the bladder and preventing leaks and which parts are vital to clamping our partners and demanding that Mercedes we keep looking at in the garage. After all, if he refuses then we can 'spit' him out and remain closed for business such is the strength of a vaginal contraction, until negotiations are going our way! Yes he can go shopping elsewhere but as every woman reads this book, and strengthens her vaginal wall, he will be spat out more than once! Give up the ghost and buy the car for the one you love.

Imagine this scenario; you are lying down and your partner is inside you - trouble is that your vaginal wall is so open and your pelvic floor so weak that it is like having a spoon stirring around in a yoghurt pot not touching the edge!

Awakening our 'core' — Discovering our trump card!

Chapter 2

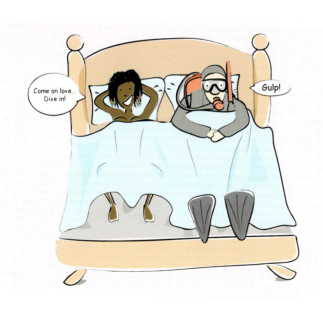

This is a common occurrence for thousands of women. When I do pelvic floor co-ordination in class, I am astonished at the amount of women that say: "Help me I am letting my husband down" or, "It does not work like that". Others may say, "I have no idea how to co-ordinate that exercise much less use it". I find it all too frightening. What must these women be doing at home? Many women even admit that their vaginal wall was never near closed to begin with and there are women in their late twenties and early thirties without children, who cannot wear a regular or mini tampon because it FALLS OUT! How scary is that! Women have said to me "so are you telling me

Awakening our 'core' — Discovering our trump card!

Chapter 2

that if my husband is inside me and I cannot feel anything that is my fault?" Or, "Could I really fix or improve it?" Many of these same women experience minor incontinence in certain situations, such as hearty laughter or running and jumping or will experience this sooner rather than later. Left unchecked, this can/will develop into an embarrassing and bigger issue.

A little food for thought here. Most of us strive to have those wonderful upper abdominals spending many hours doing hundreds of sit ups in our quest for a flatter stomach. Did you realize when the upper abdominals become overly strong to their lower abdominal partners they can cause greater pressure on the lower abdominals making their job even harder and is another cause of pelvic floor dysfunction and incontinence, especially when lifting, pushing or pulling/pounding (running) which places increased pressure through the abdominals and further loads the already weakened lower abs and pelvic floor! Watch that!

Many of us will go to class where the buzz words are "set your 'core'" but with so many courses on the market and not so many doing in-depth study, people are being told to 'tighten the

Awakening our 'core' — Discovering our trump card!

Chapter 2

abdominals' or 'set the core' when they are not really aware of the exact role the stabilizers play. The upper abdominals (or Rectus Abdomens) are a stabilizer under dynamic load, such as an American footballer or a rugby player being charged at from behind. Where great load or force is needed this muscle would have to work to protect the upper back and head from trauma. The waistline (oblique) is a stabilizer and support for the rib cage and protects them. It helps to anchor the hips and control movements like tossing a ball or sudden movements like reaching out to return a backhand in tennis, or stopping a child from unexpectedly running into the street. In these instances we would need the use of these stabilizers but we are being misled into engaging them as a unit, which is not their function for most of the exercises or everyday activities we do.

Man at the bar

I want you to focus from the umbilicus down. When we activate our core we need to re-educate the brain to breathe from our tummy (diaphragmatically). Most of us have been taught to do the short shallow breathing or as I say 'the man at the bar' breath, you know the one you do when someone catches your

Awakening our 'core' – Discovering our trump card!

Chapter 2

eye. Your diaphragm is drawn in and up and you elevate your chest so as to look taller and leaner through the trunk. A good way to see if you are not breathing diaphragmatically is by standing in front of a mirror and watching for any excessive movement with the shoulders, or the chest expanding and elevating - this is short shallow breathing. When we inhale through the nose it is like pumping air into a ball. The shoulders and chest should remain still and the diaphragm (tummy) should expand. As we exhale we should draw the umbilicus (belly button) in and slightly up toward the spine. Now if you draw in too tightly

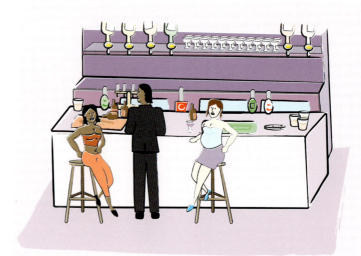

Awakening our 'core' – Discovering our trump card!

Chapter 2

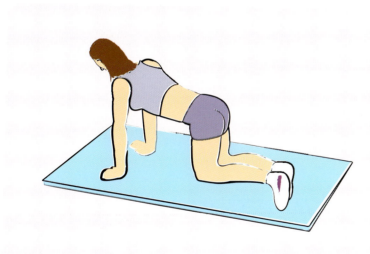

fig 1

you will feel a restriction in the chest, which means you have engaged the oblique also and are depressing the rib cage. You have drawn in too far. Allow the umbilicus to release a little until the diaphragm is free, so that you will be able to breathe freely with the 'core' set. Remember if you inhale and draw in, this is an unnatural movement. We have retrained our bodies to do in the quest to look taller and leaner. If you put air into a balloon it will inflate, the same is true of the lungs and diaphragm.

A good way to begin to activate the lower abdominals (TVA) is to get down on all fours *fig 1*. The key points here are

Awakening our 'core' — Discovering our trump card!

Chapter 2

to ensure that the hands are directly below the shoulders and the knees directly below the hips. Inhale in this position and the gravitational pull from the viscera (internal organs of the body - the intestines for example) is felt, the stretch reflex is activated to switch on the TVA by drawing the umbilicus towards the spine and slightly upward. The last and important point here is to keep the back neutral - do not excessively tip the pelvis (dip lower back) or overly round the low back. Once you master this (do 10 x 10 sec hold) progress to standing tummy vacuums.

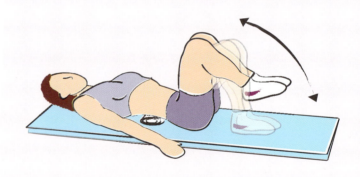

fig 2

Awakening our 'core' – Discovering our trump card!

Chapter 2

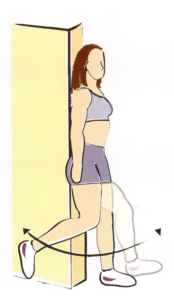

fig 3

Another exercise that is good for our lower abdominals and limb co-ordination is to lie on your back and place fingers under the back (at L3 disc on lumbar spine) directly behind the bellybutton, with your fingertips touching. A firm but slight pressure should be maintained on the fingers throughout the exercise. Keeping the head, neck and shoulders relaxed, inhale and dome the tummy and then draw the umbilicus inward as you exhale. Practice some rhythmic breathing whilst holding this position before adding movement 'from the hip area' lifting the feet. First only lift until parallel to the floor and then integrate lower abs with the TVA by lifting the leg to a right ankle and lowering, progressing

Awakening our 'core' – Discovering our trump card!

Chapter 2

on to lifting and lowering both at the same time. Whilst you are doing all these variations what you are trying to achieve is stability through the lower back. You should not be doming/swelling the tummy as you lift and lower and the pressure applied to the fingers should remain constant.

With my clients I use a blood pressure cuff *fig 2* (usually placed around the upper of the arm to measure blood pressure) under the lower back instead of the fingers. By pumping to a certain point (40ml) I create a natural cushion between the lower back and the floor. Then when the pelvis is tilted to apply the light but firm pressure

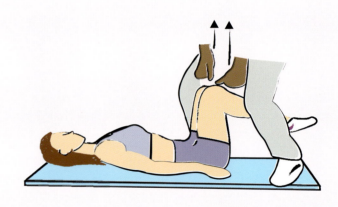

fig 4

Awakening our 'core' — Discovering our trump card!

Chapter 2

the needle will raise (70ml) and give all the indication of stability by remaining as close to the set goal as possible. The penultimate test for the TVA is to do this exercise standing against a wall *fig 3*. You really do need a blood pressure cuff for this one. This will ensure that you can truly activate the TVA while standing and moving the legs (massive load here on pelvic area and stabilizers. This means you have a greater sense of coordination and strength in this arena). There is a high carry over from this exercise to many of the ways in which we make love, as well as everyday situations. It is in these positions that we can really enhance the way in which we increase the pleasure for our partners and especially for ourselves, and the levels and lengths of orgasm.

The final LA exercise is to incorporate a raising and lowering of the thighs at a right angle using the TVA *fig 4*. Lying on your back you have a right angle at the hips and knees. Activate the TVA and then use this and the TVA to elevate the knees by a couple of inches toward the ceiling. (Ref: Scientific Core Conditioning - Paul Chek C.H.E.K. Institute).

Spend at least four weeks mastering these exercises and incorporating them into your everyday life or current

Awakening our 'core' – Discovering our trump card!

Chapter 2

exercise program. Once you are there it is time to learn all the pelvic floor exercises before you try and coordinate them together! - We are on our way!

I quoted the title of this book to a few male friends of mine to ask whether they thought they would they pick the book up off the shelf if they saw it. The answer was yes. Many men found the title hilarious but all were quick to add: "I believe it could. You women do not understand just what you have down there". As another man put it: "Many women are literally sitting on a goldmine". I bet many of us did not realize that this was the case.

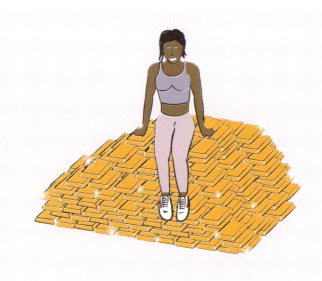

So what's so special about our Pelvic Floor?

Chapter 3

This poor little muscle is so overlooked and yet controls so much of what we take for granted and enjoy. Why don't we have the education from school days that takes care of this for all us females? We learn about sexually transmitted infections and how easy it is to get pregnant, History teaches us about great leaders of people who have influenced change in our lives, how mathematics can influence us should we choose to become mathematicians, scientists or computer technicians. We learn how to pronounce our 'P's' and 'Q's'. Yet we are never told that as females, just holding our urine all day can be detrimental to our pelvic floor later on. No one mentions the word 'continence' in the context of pelvic floor, which would at least tell us we have good bladder control and can stay dry, and that 'incontinence' is an involuntary loss of control of the bladder at inconvenient times that can prove embarrassing. Very few midwifes tell us that if we neglect the pelvic floor after natural childbirth we could run the risk of having our very own Channel Tunnel. The trauma of childbirth on the pelvic floor through natural childbirth can be major if the muscle is not re-conditioned. And, many young women who experience sexual abuse as children can have long-term implications on their pelvic floor function. As pelvic floor dysfunction

So what's so special about our Pelvic Floor?

Chapter 3

seems to only be linked to childbirth, continence pads are used in place of reconditioning exercises, but the re-education of the Pelvic Floor is missing. Many other factors can affect the working of the pelvic floor. The list below is just a few of them:

- Low estrogen states
- Menopause
- Ageing
- Constipation and/or Chronic Cough
- Being Overweight
- Drugs
- Spinal Problems
- Catheters
- Brain Damage
- Stroke, Parkinson's disease and diabetes.

(reference: *Women's Waterworks - curing incontinence by Dr Pauline Chiarelli*).

There are other serious pelvic floor issues that are beyond this book and for these one would need to seek qualified and professional advice. Let me list some below:

Sexual dysfunctions

- Vaginal Hypertonia - dyspareunia (overactive muscle spasm painful during penetration)
- Vaginismus. (painful penetration)

So what's so special about our Pelvic Floor?

Chapter 3

> "The vaginal wall is a bag of muscle and unconditioned muscles do not function properly"

- Vaginal Hypotonia . (no muscles tone, no reactions)
- Orgasmic Dysfunction
- Genitourinary Pathology and Sexuality
- Low libido
- Sexual aversion disorder.

Stress incontinence

- Condition of perineal body during vaginal birth
- Micturition reflex
- Stop test
- Strength and condition of the Levator ani
- Parturition
- Type I and Type II fibres
- Sexual trauma and abuse
- Inner unit shut down.

Ageing is quite significant. As we age our muscles shrink away and we lose flexibility and range of movement. Remember the vaginal wall is a bag of muscle and unconditioned muscles do not function properly. The pelvic floor acts as a support for the abdominal contents. If it is weak its ability to hold them is greatly decreased. Constipation and chronic cough also causes immense amounts of pressure over time because of the consistent intra-abdominal pressure bearing down every time you cough or strain to empty the bowels. Remember none of these things take

So what's so special about our Pelvic Floor?

Chapter 3

effect until you have destroyed the strength of the pelvic floor. With the transverse as the walls of a cylinder that offer no support, the contents just keep dropping until they fall through. The worse case scenario is a prolapsed bladder - hanging out of the vaginal wall! It does happen and often, ask a gynecologist! Another adage is sexual dysfunction, which was defined by the World Health Organisation in 1992 as: 'the various ways in which an individual is unable to participate in a sexual relationship as he or she would like'.

(Ref: *Make It or Fake It by Dr Grace Dorey PhD MCSP*)

Awakening the Pelvic Floor

Chapter 4

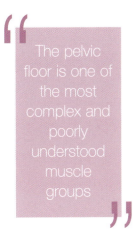

> The pelvic floor is one of the most complex and poorly understood muscle groups

What I would like to do firstly is re-introduce you to your vagina. You need to know the muscles that are responsible for keeping the bladder under control and the feeling of a need to leak, and the muscles that are responsible for making that man of yours scream and moan!

In the following paragraphs I have included the dictionary definitions of technical terms for the muscles in the vagina so it will make sense to us all. The brackets that follow these words give their definition.

The pelvic floor is a very 'responsible' muscle that most of us have no appreciation for until we begin to leak when we laugh, sneeze or cough, or find painful with deep penetration during sex. The pelvic floor is a collection of tissue that spans the opening within the bony pelvis. It lies at the bottom of the abdominal pelvic cavity and forms a supporting layer for the abdominal and pelvic viscera (the internal organs of the body, such as the intestines). The urethra, bladder and supporting structures of the pelvis are all part of the pelvic floor. The pelvic floor is one of the most complex and poorly understood muscle groups in the body. This may be because it is internal so the focus is overlooked until there is a problem. Our drive for aesthetics

Awakening the Pelvic Floor

Chapter 4

does not include this, as we do not see it; although now we have the new 'designer vaginas' we still have no focus on its importance of function. Levator ani (Levator - a muscle that helps to lift the body part to which it is attached) must support the weight of the pelvic contents and resist increased intra-abdominal pressure (pressure from inside the muscle) which can come about in our everyday activities - bending over to pick up a heavy object, sneezing, laughing etc. If you think there is not much activity within the wall the next time you laugh, put your hands on your tummy, or when you sneeze focus on how your abdominal wall responds. Both the resting tone and voluntary contraction are important for pelvic support as just mentioned in the examples above.

Pelvic floor exercise would increase the strength of the urogenital (relating to, or involving, the organs of the urinary tract and the reproductive organs when considered together), sphincter (a circular band of muscle that surrounds an opening or passage in the body and narrows or closes the opening by contracting) a striated muscle which is under some volitional (the act of will distinguished from the intended

Awakening the Pelvic Floor

Chapter 4

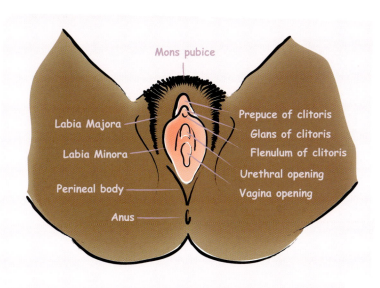

physical movement, it causes) control. The function of the pubovisceral muscle (pubococcygeus located as part of a muscular pelvic floor diaphragm across the outlet of the bony pelvis - one of the two muscles that form the levator ani) is to pull the rectum, vagina and urethra forward towards the pubic bones, compressing their lumens (openings). Thus increasing the strength of this muscle group would increase closure of these structures.

Part of a quote given to us at church one Sunday was "It's not what you read but what you remember that makes you learned". When it comes to our vagina and we are quoted 'vestibular bulb'

Awakening the Pelvic Floor

Chapter 4

and 'Bartholin's gland' without identification for which part of the vagina this is, then it has gone over our heads and we either do not understand or we forget what it is we are told. If we know that 'inner labia' means the lips and that the 'vestibular bulbs' are the erectile tissue on either side of the urethra (urethra being the short tube above the vagina that connects the bladder to the outer side of the body) which swell during sexual excitement and contribute to the tightness felt around the penis at the vaginal entrance, along with stimulation of the clitoris, we are more inclined to remember. The Bartholin's gland is the greater vestibular glands which are mucous glands the size of a pea at the opening either side of the vaginal entrance. They produce mucoid secretions during sexual arousal (juice). The muscle in our vagina (a canal approximately 7-15cm in length), is involuntary and lined with this mucous membrane. During sexual arousal this involuntary muscle relaxes as the vagina widens and dilates, and expands and the lubrication fluid is released. The periurethral glans - peri meaning mobile - is a triangular membrane that moves in and out during penile

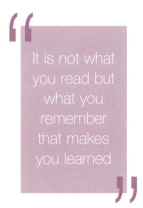

" It is not what you read but what you remember that makes you learned "

Awakening the Pelvic Floor

Chapter 4

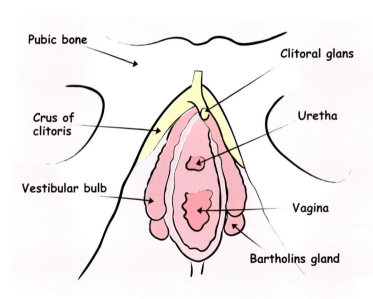

trusting. (Ref: Make It or Fake It by Dr Grace Dorey PhD MCSP).

As most of us are or have been sexually active, visualization allows us to understand and get it right - so lets use the cartoon sketches and language to understand how we make this part of the body look good, protect us from embarrassment and make our partners want for nothing! (Great sex yeah!) (Ref: What your mother never told you about S-E-X, Hilda Hutcherson).

Why do I find this subject so fascinating? I may teach it in jest, but I get bombarded with requests for help to redress the issue. I am no

Awakening the Pelvic Floor

Chapter 4

medical doctor, it really does stem from what was mentioned in the first paragraph. Most medical books are very technical and written in Latin. At the end of the day, people just want to know what to do. The more I talk about it, the more I find out that this is not an issue associated with post natal women. On the contrary, there are too many women who have not experienced the changing of the vaginal passage because of childbirth, yet have many issues or reasons for being in the same position. Gather a group of women together over a couple of drinks, and bring it up in conversation. I guarantee that at least one will have minor incontinence and another will have a big gap downstairs that leaves them wondering 'what he really feels like'! There is no quick fix here, it can be a slow process - but if you think of yourself as having years ahead of you and plenty of time to practice and co-ordinate then you have nothing to worry about. The main issue is how you prioritise your time and practice. Not the act of sex but the 'solo' exercise. It takes about 350 repetitions for a movement to become an automatic pattern that the brain will recognize. In order to get to a state of automacy you must put the reps in.

> So armed with this information, let us now focus on our pelvic floor exercises.

Awakening the Pelvic Floor

Chapter 4

Remember though, if you train in a faulty training pattern, then it could take up to 5,000 repetitions to undo it and then a further 350 good ones to make it another 'motor engram' - automatic pattern! An example of this is when you are learning to use the pelvic floor with too much use of the butt. This is faulty because you are not identifying pelvic floor alone but rather that the butt leads the movement.

So armed with this information, let us now focus on our pelvic floor exercises.

We want to be able to link together our lower abdominals and pelvic floor.

Firstly, do the following exercises without first setting your lower abdominals and then repeat them and set your 'core' - lower abdominals and feel the difference in the intensity and contraction. You are on your way to full function. What we want to be able to do is feel the contraction start from within the outer lips of the vaginal wall and then feel the difference in the depth when we first set out TVA - trust me, a big difference - (remember they work on the same neurological loop), I am repeating this to emphasis the importance of the relationship. If you go onto a search engine to find

Awakening the Pelvic Floor

Chapter 4

information on this you will find thousands of sites all with very technical "I needed a dictionary to decipher" stuff.

Stand with your legs apart. Imagine you want to open the vagina. Try and push down gently and feel the pelvic floor drop and open. Did you feel that? Please do not tell me no: Damn yours is open already! We are in trouble. In its relaxed state it should be elevated and closed. You should feel it move.

I want you to visualize that you are standing up and are desperate to go to the toilet. You need to stop yourself

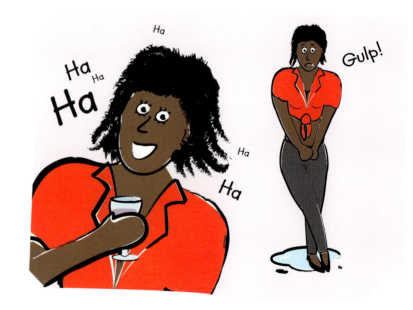

Awakening the Pelvic Floor

Chapter 4

but you must not squeeze from the butt first. Close your eyes and focus completely on your vaginal wall - imagine you are trying to close the lips together and reverse the urine back up into the bladder - a bit like drinking up through a straw. The base of the straw is inside the vagina, and the top of the straw coming out of the belly button. How deep was the contraction? As you tried to squeeze tighter how much of the contractions did you feel in your butt? And what about the abdominal wall? OK, quite a lot. I want you to repeat this and stop as soon as the contraction elsewhere seems to dominate. Now set your TVA and then repeat this exercise. Was the contraction deeper within the vaginal wall without too much intervention from the butt? Place your hand between the pubic bone and the belly button and imagine a straw runs from inside the vaginal wall to the belly button. You need to drink up and feel the movement under the hand. The squeeze must be led from the front first. If you focus from behind first you will develop a faulty training pattern and we already know how much work that can take to undo. Your body always migrates towards its position of strength and if you train your pelvic floor this way you lose. Read the scenario on the next page.

Awakening the Pelvic Floor

Chapter 4

Jimmy Choo

Jimmy Choo shoes are wonderful and very expensive, so it would be a crying shame to sneeze and wet them. Imagine you are out in the outback in your Jimmy Choos', as you do, and you are desperate to go to the toilet. Off you run into a bush and squat to pee. Now if you do not sit your hip back behind your heels and keep your chest forward and the shoulders up to the sky, albeit at a slight forward angle, you will pee on those shoes. So you squat low and well, the thing is, just as you are about to pee, you look down and realize you are crouching over a snake that is just starting to stir. You need to get up but your pelvic floor is weak and your core is asleep. A shock like that could make you lose a little liquid and that's it, game over! But this is not you! You have got to grips with setting your core and would do that even just to hold the squat and not stress the back. So I want you to focus on your vaginal lips, and try and draw them together as you drink up. Yes, you will get a pull from behind (that's because the levator ani is at work here and remember it pulls the rectum too), but make sure the contraction starts from front to back and not back to front. Great, that's engaged so now the hip extensors are activated = your butt

Awakening the Pelvic Floor

Chapter 4

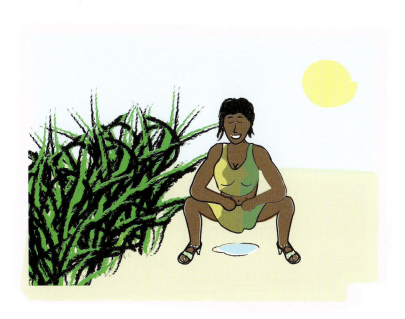

and hamstring and up you come, lid closed no leaks and you can escape, the snake just stirring! It is very hard to engage the pelvic floor when the legs are apart but it is vital to your rehab program. Otherwise if you can only engage the floor with the legs together how on earth is he ever going to get in? Men can do this same position and draw up through their testicles – it is quite enlightening for them also, and a lovely feeling for us – seen it, experienced it! Remember men; this assists in prolonging the act and offsets premature ejaculation.

Now we are on the floor, face downwards *fig 5*. You need to try and

Awakening the Pelvic Floor

Chapter 4

rest on the inside of the knees on the floor and place the soles of the feet together as close to the bottom as possible. You have opened up your vagina fully so the contraction is much harder, but this is a pelvic floor rehab exercise used in hospitals. What I want you to do first is in/exhale and set the belly button (that alone is hard to do and maintain in this position) now focus on the vaginal wall and try to close the lips and drink up. It is hard, but definitely a good one as in this position the butt can hardly play. Twenty-one repetitions later you are ready to move on (use your imagination and put this

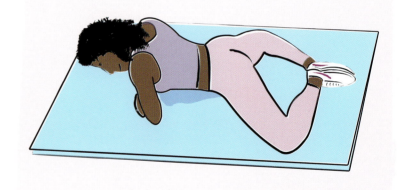

fig 5

Awakening the Pelvic Floor

Chapter 4

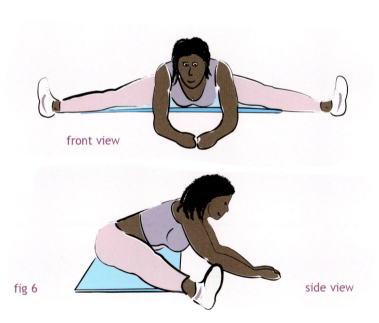

front view

fig 6   side view

scenario and your strengthened pelvic floor into your bedroom = two very happy people.

Bouncing butts and laughter

Sit yourself round in the straddle position *fig 6 front and side*. This is one of the most amusing of all the exercises I do in my master class. Take your legs out east and west and try to rotate the pelvis under so you are literally sitting on the base of the vagina, (really need to be able to forward tilt the pelvis and release the lower back). Once again the wall is open. Set the core first and then try and close the vagina. What we are looking for here is great control and

Awakening the Pelvic Floor

Chapter 4

rhythm, so that the butt cheeks start dancing - it is a great sight to see 90+ women trying to bounce their butts on the floor whilst engaging their pelvic floor - one hand forward and that can spark a conversation or the beginning of a request for something that should not be rejected!

Another set of exercises is to lie on your back with the legs apart and try to draw the thighs together using the vaginal wall first, followed through by the inner thighs. Still lying on your back, put your legs at 90 degrees and set your lower abs. Begin to lower and lift one leg at a time (pos as *fig 2*). On the downward phase close the vaginal wall first. Try first to engage the pelvic floor by drawing the lips together just inside the vaginal wall as if to close around a straw and then have a drink up to the belly button. Try to ensure you are closing from inside the vagina and not closing the anal passage, and then lower a leg, release at the bottom and then return to the start. Then try the whole exercise in reverse. Lower the leg, close the vaginal wall and then try to lift the leg keeping everything engaged. Harder? Initially try eight to ten repetitions of each and once you have mastered that then try to keep the wall engaged whilst lifting and then

Awakening the Pelvic Floor

Chapter 4

lowering. You can increase the intensity of the lift by altering the position or height of the leg from the floor. The closer the feet are to the floor, the greater the load and therefore there will be an activation of the rectus abdomens (upper abdominals). Use regular rhythmic breathing. If you find this hard to begin with bring the knees back to slightly above/behind the hips.

There are a multitude of ways to test out the strength of the vaginal wall so that no matter what you are doing you never leak, and no matter how you express yourself with your partner you can use it optimally.

Just before we go any further, we need to see where we are at and put these tools - our lower abdominals and pelvic floor - to the test. Many of my clients say that their vaginal wall is like Blackwall Tunnel and could hold nothing in. If you have been doing the exercises in this book over a period of time, then you will have conditioning in your abdominal wall and pelvic floor. Read on...this is a great test for you.

Along came Gynaflex

Chapter 5

Just when you thought you had won the war on the unconditioned pelvic floor along comes the Gynaeflex! This gadget is patented and comes in six strengths for good reason also! It is the thigh master for the vagina! Once again, I was stunned at the amount of work I still needed to do to strengthen the muscles of my pelvic floor. It really was a "let's start at the very beginning"! scenario. I have tried no.4, and initially, I struggled, (bragging I was that good), albeit for a week or so. A program lasting twelve weeks, with this gadget, will seriously improve the strength of your pelvic floor. This is a well designed, conditioning program for the muscles inside the vaginal wall! The Gynaeflex machine allows you to immediately focus on the pelvic floor, and its design lets you know the moment you use too much recruitment from the butt or lower abdominals. Do not get me wrong, I want you to co-ordinate the pelvic with abdominal, but you must know first how to switch it on without using the butt as its switch.

As I explained earlier the whole body works as one kinetic chain, but with faulty training patterns we tend to recruit the muscles from our bottoms first and therefore have secondary

Along came Gynaflex

Chapter 5

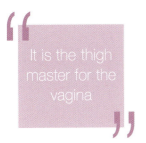

" It is the thigh master for the vagina "

recruitment from the vaginal wall and pelvic floor. This is why we find it so hard to co-ordinate it into our exercise program, our focus is all backwards.

I strongly recommend that once you have done all the exercises mentioned earlier in this book and feel confident about where you are and the strength you have in your pelvic floor, put it to the test by investing in a set of Gynaeflex. The truth will tell.

OK, so you have done your exercises, you have purchased and used your Gynaeflex, now you are ready for one last test.

Mines' a cotton bud please

If you are between relationships this is a great test for you also. They say size is everything. I beg to differ. Get out your cotton bud when you are just about to head for the showers – this exercise is private! Set your lower abdominals – close the lid on your cylinder. Now draw the lips of the vaginal wall together and 'drink through our straw'. Insert the cotton bud halfway. If your wall is tight enough you will feel it glide in against the vaginal wall. Start to squat, move the legs around sideways, forward, backwards etc and the bud should remain still. When you have finished

Along came Gynaflex

Chapter 5

fooling around remove the bud and you should feel it leave! Got it. Size is not everything, tightness and good co-ordination is! Get practicing. "Coming darling, I'm just doing a little warm up first".

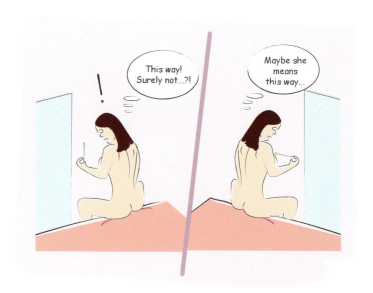

Taking the car for a test drive

Conclusion

I am finished. What can I say? I am writing as I speak in master class and lectures. I hope you have found this a pleasurable read, and you will do the exercises - after all what have you got to lose? Women come to me everyday and want great abs, thighs and butts. As women we never think of our arms, upper back or vaginal wall. Let me add this last scenario that I give all women in class.

I can work the areas you want and make them look good, hell I have done that over time on myself. I though am a head to toe person, so I leave nothing to chance. Most women will not mention their arms or upper back. As one client told me recently once she reaches 40 she will cover up those areas forever, and wear clothing appropriate to her age! My answer is this. We have worked consistently only on the areas you wanted. You have the desired results and now you are invited to the Ball, a major event for you. Everything you worked on you 'cover' with that wonderful evening dress you have just invested so much money in. It's beautiful, and strapless. Thing is, everything you forgot to work on you leave exposed. So you squeezed yourself into your size ten, and that excess body fat around the shoulders hangs out and when you wave to your friend, that excess body fat at the back

Taking the car for a test drive

Conclusion

of the arm keeps vibrating some ten seconds later! Scary!

Now imagine also a great end to a perfect evening. You have been dating this man forever and you finally are ready to express yourself – or that dress was your wedding dress and you are going to consummate your marriage. Everything we worked on you hide. You know you leak when you laugh, sneeze, jump, run or cough.

You know you have no tone in your vaginal muscles yet you chose to ignore it. All you wanted was great looking abs and thighs. Are you really confident this will be the mind blowing experience you dreamed it would be? Betty Wright once sung a fantastic ballad: "Tonight is the night that you make me a woman". If you leave nothing to chance you can never be disappointed. It's a muscle - why not use it? Happy exercising.

> "You know that when you laugh, sneeze, run, jump or cough you leak"

Glossary

Abdominal
The muscles that form the wall of the abdomen; our midsection of the trunk.

Blackwall Tunnel
Four-lane underground tunnel linking North and South of London.

Bladder
The organ (sac) inside the pelvic area used for storing urine.

Bartholins glands
Part of the greater vestibular gland the size of a pea just outside the opening of the vagina.

Clitoris
Organ of erectile tissue at the top of the vagina, which becomes swollen when correctly stimulated and can result in orgasm.

Continence
The ability to prevent involuntary urination and or bowel movements; it is also the ability to control physical (especially sexual) impulses allowing for self-restraint, moderation or abstinence.

Diaphragm
A curved muscular membrane that separates the abdomen from the area around the lungs.

Glossary

Incontinence
The inability to control involuntary urination or bowel movements; a lack of sexual restraint or self-control - literally a lack of moderation of an action or emotion.

Kinesiology
The study of the mechanics of motion with respect to human anatomy. It allows for muscle testing that reveals and corrects musculoskeletal imbalances and identifies food sensitivities.

Levator
A muscle that helps to lift the body part to which it is attached.

Levator Ani
Two part muscle (front part also known as pubococcygeus - sling that pulls the rectum, vagina and urethra anteriorly towards the pubic bones, the second part is known as the illiococcygeus - a horizontal sheet that assists in the support of the pelvic viscera.

Multifidus
Lying just under the erector spine, this muscle has many lobe shaped segments and is the true stabilizer of the lower back.

Neurological
The function of the nervous system affecting both nerve and muscle tissue.

Glossary

Oblique
Slanting muscles in the midsection, which support the rib cage.

Rectus Abdominal
Rectus being any straight muscle, is the upper part of the abdominal structure.

Stabilization
The act or process of keeping something in place; maintaining balance.

Tran versus
Lower section of the abdominal lying and extending crosswise.

Umbilicus
Navel/belly button.

Urethra
The short tube above the vagina that connects the bladder to the outer side of the body.

Vestibular bulbs
The erectile tissue that becomes swollen during sexual arousal.

Viscera
The internal organs in the body, especially those of the abdomen such as the intestines.

References and further reading

Paul Chek Seminars
Scientific Core Conditioning
Equal but not the Same – considerations for training females
Movement that matters
www.paulchekseminars.com

Dr Grace Dorey PhD MCSP
Make It or Fake It

Dr Pauline Chiarelli
Women's Waterworks - curing incontinence

Dr Hilda Hutcherson
What Your Mother Never Told You About S-E-X

B Schussler, J Laycock
Pelvic Floor Re-education

Specialist Therapists:

ACA Association for Continence Advice
102a Astra House
Arklow Road
New Cross
LONDON SE14 6EB
tel: 020 8692 4680
email: info@aca.uk.com

ACPWH Association of Chartered Physiotherapists in Women's Health
C/o the Chartered Society of Physiotherapy
14 Bedford Row
LONDON WC1R 4ED
tel: 020 7306 6666
website: http://www.womentsphysio.com

For therapists in your area, enter 'continence therapists' into an online search engine.

About the author

Jenni Russell has won the title "Britain's Fittest Woman" after winning the British Ultrafit Championships three times. She also won Channel Five's 'Dessert Forges' in 2000.

An athlete first, Jenni runs her own personal training consultancy. Her specialized field is 'core' abs/back conditioning, focusing also on its relationship to pelvic floor incontinence and sexual function. She presents workshops at fitness weekends and holidays (for Mbrace Fitness Ltd), and has also given a presentation on Transverse and Pelvic Floor relationship at the North and West London Faculty of the Royal College of General Practitioners Research and Innovation Conference 2003. Her contribution to the industry was recognized last October (2004) at a Celebratory Dinner in Park Lane, London, where she won the Training Category award of the European Federation of Black Women Business Owners.

This book has been Jenni's 'baby' for the last three years. After much laughter and deliberation, and after listening to clients concerns in this area, Jenni finally decided that this book was needed. Once she was comfortable enough to expose a bit of herself, she put together this fun filled user-friendly book, which will

About the author

benefit all females - aesthetically, 'continent', sexually active or otherwise.

Look out for her DVD's: 'The Stability Ball is my Best Friend' - a beginners guide to building confidence and respect for the ball & 'The Next Level' - Advanced Stability Ball Training aimed at the personal trainer or studio teacher who would like to add a little more than the basic exercises we see the ball being used for every day but lack the confidence or vision as too just what the ball can be used for. Both are available to order via her website www.shapeyourthang.com (www.jennirussell.com coming soon).

In addition to honoring her commitments to her clients and the private health clubs where she teaches, Jenni also presents master classes and workshops, and is mother to her beautiful, well-balanced and gifted son, Jourdan-Reiss.

Special thanks

My first thanks, has to be to God, who makes all things possible and I give thanks to be a part of his kingdom. A special thank you for my son, Jourdan-Reiss Russell, for your patience and support whilst I have been running around doing these workshops, and getting together the information needed for this book. As young as you are it was sheer delight to see your face light up when you presented the draft to the family...Granddad's face was a picture. I really love you. I want to thank my parents, Mr and Mrs Russell, for all your patience whilst I made my excuses for not working so that I could write.

I thank Paul Chek for telling me to put it into words in the first place, and then taking the time to read it. Thanks for your continuing education.

A special thank you has to go to Peter and Claudette. You both saw the passion in me and had faith enough to provide the resource needed to 'Make my Dream a Reality'. My payback is to be able to see the vision in that next person who has the drive but needs the opportunity to be realized.

Last, but by no means least, I would like to thank Alison and David Key for all your help and support. Thank you Alison for coming to my workshop in

Special thanks

Wales and finding it enlightening enough for you to want to help me with this book. Thank you to your wonderful husband, David (Stud Agent David to me), for working on all my pictures (not just the book, but my biography portfolio and DVD artwork) - they are great! Your mum Pauline, my 'other mother', is an inspiration. Your family has been very supportive and I love you all for that. Lets hope the Mercedes you get is the one you want!